TRIM THE TUMMY: WELLNESS WISDOM FOR A LEANER YOU

Your Blueprint to a Healthier, Happier Waistline

BY ALEXANDER ELY

contents

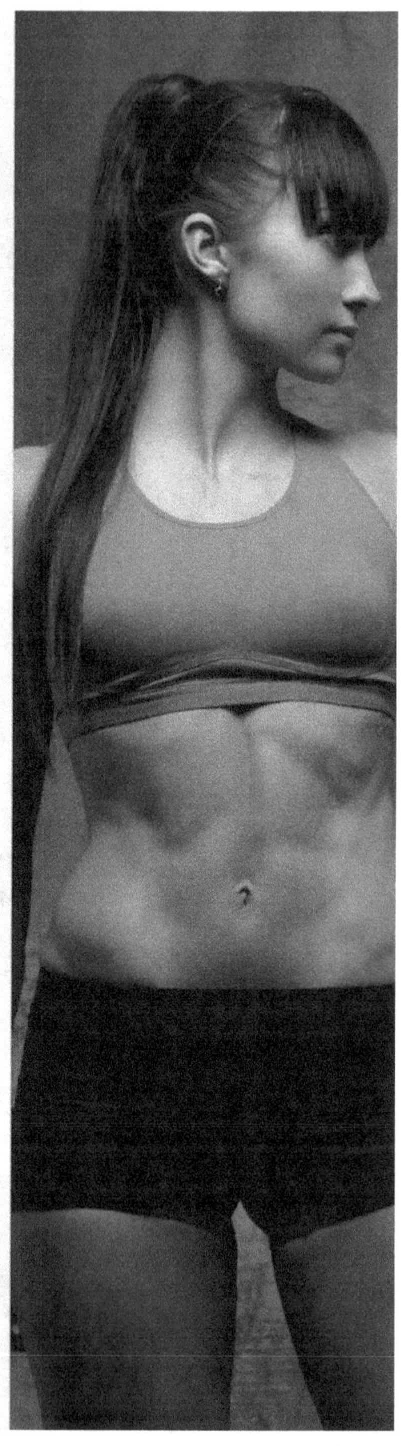

Introduction

Have you ever felt overwhelmed by the countless health fads and fitness trends, all promising a leaner midsection? You're not alone. But what if there was a more profound, holistic approach that went beyond mere aesthetics and dove deep into overall well-being? "Trim the Tummy: Wellness Wisdom for a Leaner You" is precisely that guide. Instead of fleeting solutions, we delve into the interconnected realms of nutrition, holistic exercises, sleep, and stress management. This isn't just about a trimmer waistline; it's about unlocking a vibrant, healthier version of yourself.

In a world saturated with quick fixes, this book stands out as your beacon to genuine wellness. We'll debunk myths, challenge the status quo, and provide actionable steps rooted in science and real-world experience. Each page is designed not just to inform, but to inspire and ignite a passion for true health. If you're ready for a transformative journey that promises more than just a leaner tummy, but a richer, more fulfilling life, then keep reading. Your path to holistic wellness starts here. Let's embark on this adventure together.

Chapter 1

THE ANATOMY OF BELLY FAT

UNDERSTANDING THE LAYERS

When we talk about belly fat, it's not just a singular, uniform layer that we're referring to. Beneath the skin, our abdominal region is a complex structure, and the fat within it is layered and varied. To truly grasp the significance of belly fat and its impact on our health, it's crucial to understand its anatomy.

VISCERAL VS. SUBCUTANEOUS FAT: MORE THAN SKIN DEEP

The fat in our body isn't all the same. Primarily, when we discuss belly fat, we're talking about two distinct types: visceral and subcutaneous. Subcutaneous Fat: This is the fat that you can pinch. It lies directly under the skin and above the abdominal muscles. Everyone has subcutaneous fat, and its amount varies from person to person. While it plays a role in storing energy and insulating the body, excessive subcutaneous fat can be a cosmetic concern for many.

Visceral Fat: Often referred to as 'deep' fat, visceral fat is stored further underneath the skin, wrapping around our vital organs like the liver, pancreas, and intestines. It's more metabolically active than subcutaneous fat, meaning it has a greater impact on bodily functions and health. You can't feel it or pinch it, but its presence is far more concerning than subcutaneous fat.

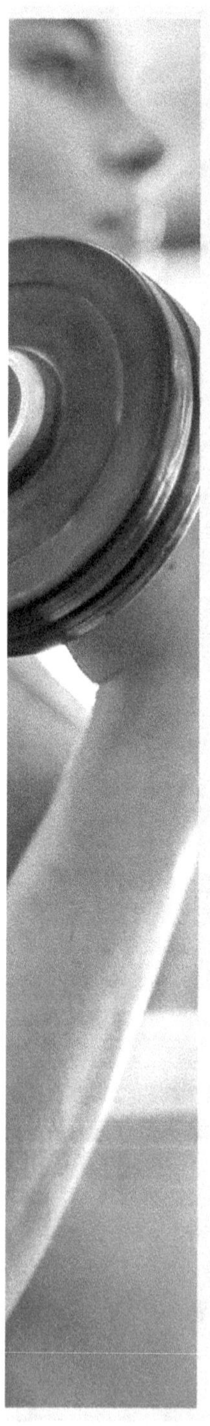

THE HEALTH IMPLICATIONS OF EXCESS BELLY FAT

While having some belly fat is natural, an excess, especially of visceral fat, can be a significant health concern. Visceral fat produces inflammatory markers, which can increase the risk of chronic diseases. Some of the health risks associated with high amounts of visceral fat include:

- **Heart Diseases**: The inflammatory substances produced can lead to heart diseases and increase cholesterol levels.
- **Type 2 Diabetes**: Visceral fat can influence insulin resistance, leading to glucose intolerance.
- **Breast and Colorectal Cancer**: There's evidence suggesting a link between visceral fat and certain types of cancer.
- **Alzheimer's Disease**: Some studies indicate that visceral fat might be a risk factor for Alzheimer's and other cognitive disorders.

Subcutaneous fat, while less harmful than visceral fat, can still pose health risks when present in excessive amounts, especially when combined with a sedentary lifestyle and poor dietary habits.

WHY THE BELLY REGION?

You might wonder, why does fat accumulate in the belly region? Genetics play a role, determining where you might store fat. Hormones, especially cortisol (a stress hormone), can influence belly fat accumulation. As we age, changes in our hormones, metabolism, and activity levels can lead to increased fat storage in the abdominal area. For women, post-menopause changes can also lead to a shift in fat storage from the hips and thighs to the belly.

Furthermore, the belly serves as a convenient and central location for the body to store energy reserves, ensuring easy access when needed. This evolutionary perspective, however, doesn't always align with our modern lifestyles, leading to an imbalance in fat storage and utilization.

In understanding the anatomy of belly fat, we're better equipped to address it. Recognizing the difference between visceral and subcutaneous fat, and the health implications of each, allows us to approach weight loss and wellness with a more informed and targeted strategy. As we progress, we'll delve deeper into holistic methods to manage and reduce belly fat, ensuring a healthier, happier you.

Chapter 2

NUTRITION NUANCES: EATING FOR A FLATTER TUMMY

THE ROLE OF MACRONUTRIENTS IN WEIGHT MANAGEMENT

Before diving into specific foods and diets, it's essential to understand the building blocks of our meals: macronutrients. These are the nutrients our bodies require in large amounts, and they play a pivotal role in energy, growth, and overall health.

Carbohydrates: Often vilified in popular diets, carbohydrates are the body's primary energy source. However, the type of carbohydrates matters. Complex carbs, like whole grains and vegetables, provide sustained energy and are packed with fiber, which aids digestion and keeps you full.

Proteins: Essential for muscle repair and growth, proteins also help in satiety. Sources include lean meats, fish, dairy, and plant-based options like beans and lentils.

Fats: Healthy fats are crucial for hormone production and nutrient absorption. Avocados, nuts, seeds, and olive oil are examples of sources that provide essential fatty acids and promote satiety.

Balancing these macronutrients in a way that aligns with your activity level and metabolic needs is key to managing weight and promoting a lean midsection.

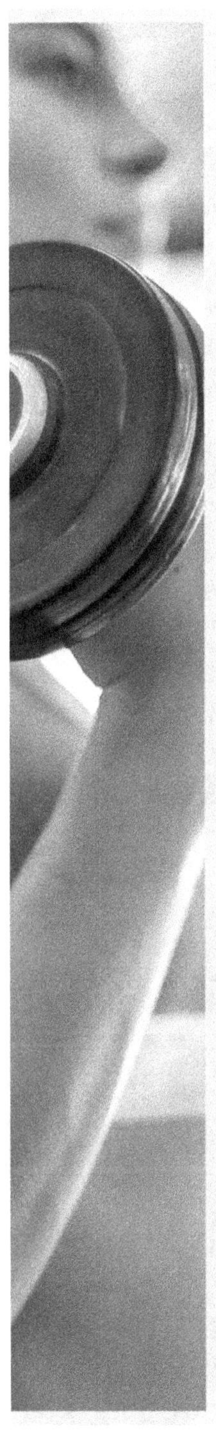

FOODS THAT PROMOTE A LEAN MIDSECTION

While no single food will magically melt away belly fat, certain foods can support metabolism, reduce bloating, and provide the nutrients needed for fat loss.
Fiber-rich Foods: Whole grains, fruits, and vegetables not only keep you full but also aid in digestion, preventing bloating and promoting gut health.

Lean Proteins: Chicken, turkey, fish, and plant-based proteins can help build muscle, which in turn boosts metabolism.

Probiotics and Fermented Foods: Yogurt, kefir, sauerkraut, and other fermented foods can improve gut health, reducing bloating and aiding digestion.

Green Tea: Some studies suggest that the catechins in green tea can aid in fat burning, especially around the belly area.

Water: While not a "food," staying hydrated helps reduce water retention and bloating, making your midsection appear leaner.

DEBUNKING DIET MYTHS

With the plethora of information available, it's easy to fall prey to diet myths. Here are a few debunked:

Myth 1: Cutting Carbs Completely is Essential for a Flat Tummy - While reducing refined carbs can help with weight loss, our bodies need carbohydrates, especially from whole, fiber-rich sources.

Myth 2: Fat Makes You Fat - Not all fats are created equal. Healthy fats, in moderation, can actually support weight loss.

Myth 3: Starvation or Extremely Low-Calorie Diets are Effective - These can slow down metabolism and lead to muscle loss, making sustainable weight loss harder.

Myth 4: "Diet Foods" are Always Better - Many low-fat or diet foods are packed with sugars or artificial sweeteners, which can hinder weight loss efforts.

Nutrition plays a pivotal role in achieving a flatter tummy. By understanding the nuances of macronutrients, incorporating foods that support a lean midsection, and steering clear of diet myths, you're setting a strong foundation for holistic health and a leaner you.

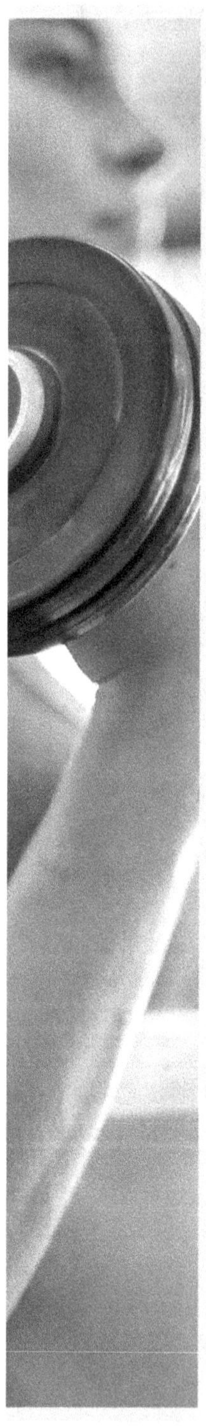

Chapter 3

THE CALORIC BALANCE: UNDERSTANDING ENERGY IN VS. ENERGY OUT

THE DANCE OF METABOLISM

At its core, metabolism is the process by which our bodies convert what we eat and drink into energy. Even when at rest, our bodies require energy for functions like breathing, circulating blood, and repairing cells. The number of calories our bodies use for these basic functions is known as the Basal Metabolic Rate (BMR).

BASICS OF METABOLISM

Metabolism isn't just about how quickly you burn calories; it's a complex interplay of chemical reactions that keep your body functioning. Factors affecting metabolism include:
- **Age**: Metabolism slows down with age.
- **Muscle Mass**: Muscle burns more calories at rest compared to fat.
- **Body Size**: Larger bodies or those with more muscle tend to burn more calories, even at rest.
- **Gender**: Men generally have a faster metabolism due to their larger muscle mass.
- **Physical Activity**: Regular activity can boost your metabolism by increasing muscle mass and the number of calories you burn.

THE ROLE OF CALORIE COUNTING

Calorie counting is a method used to track the number of calories consumed and expended, aiming to create a deficit for weight loss or a surplus for weight gain. The principle is simple:

- **Energy In**: This refers to the calories you take in from food and drink.
- **Energy Out**: This is the number of calories your body uses for bodily functions and physical activity.

To lose weight, energy out should exceed energy in. Conversely, to gain weight, energy in should be greater than energy out.

However, while calorie counting can be an effective tool, it's not the only factor in weight management. The type of calories consumed matters immensely.

QUALITY OVER QUANTITY: NUTRIENT-DENSE VS. CALORIE-DENSE FOODS

All calories are not created equal. The source of your calories plays a significant role in how your body processes them and the nutritional benefits you derive.

- **Nutrient-dense Foods**: These are foods that have a high nutrient content relative to their caloric content. Examples include vegetables, fruits, lean meats, and whole grains. They provide essential vitamins, minerals, and other beneficial compounds that support overall health.
- **Calorie-dense Foods**: These foods have a high caloric content relative to their nutrient content. Examples include sugary drinks, fast foods, and many processed snacks. While they provide energy, they often lack essential nutrients and can lead to overconsumption of calories.

By focusing on nutrient-dense foods, you not only support your weight management goals but also ensure that your body receives the vital nutrients it needs for optimal function.

In conclusion, understanding the balance between energy in and energy out is fundamental in the journey to a leaner midsection. By grasping the basics of metabolism, recognizing the role of calorie counting, and prioritizing nutrient-dense foods, you're setting the stage for sustainable and healthy weight management.

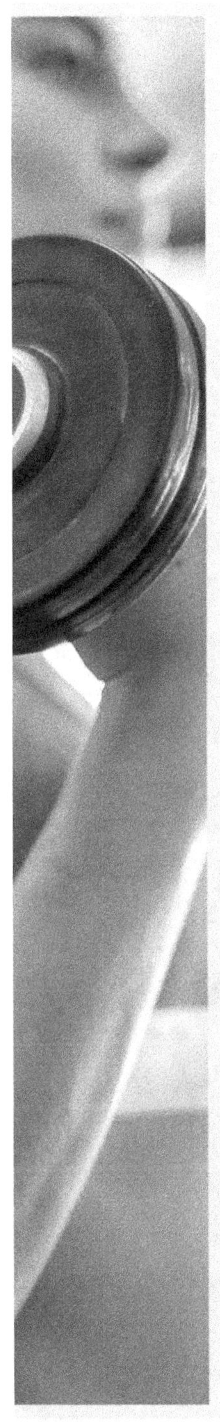

Chapter 4

CARDIOVASCULAR COMMITMENT: HEART-PUMPING PATHS TO FAT LOSS

THE HEARTBEAT OF FITNESS

Cardiovascular exercise, often simply termed as 'cardio', is the rhythmic pulse of any fitness regimen. It involves exercises that increase your heart rate, pumping oxygen-rich blood to working muscles, thereby enhancing the efficiency of your cardiovascular system.

BENEFITS OF CARDIOVASCULAR EXERCISES

Cardio is not just about burning calories; its benefits are manifold:
- **Heart Health**: Regular cardio strengthens the heart, enabling it to pump blood more efficiently, reducing the risk of heart diseases.
- **Improved Lung Capacity**: Cardio exercises increase lung capacity, ensuring better oxygen supply to the body.
- **Mood Enhancement**: Cardio releases endorphins, the body's natural painkillers, which can elevate mood and reduce stress.
- **Increased Metabolism**: Post-cardio, the body experiences an elevated calorie burn rate, known as the afterburn effect or Excess Post-exercise Oxygen Consumption (EPOC).
- **Enhanced Immune Response**: Regular cardiovascular activity can bolster the body's immune defenses.

HIIT VS. STEADY-STATE CARDIO: WHICH IS BETTER?

The debate between High-Intensity Interval Training (HIIT) and steady-state cardio is ongoing, but understanding their unique benefits can help you make an informed choice:

- **HIIT**: This involves short bursts of high-intensity exercises followed by rest or low-intensity periods. Benefits include shorter workout durations, increased calorie burn even after the workout (EPOC), and potential muscle preservation.
- **Steady-State Cardio**: This involves longer durations of moderate-intensity exercises, like jogging or cycling. Benefits include being easier on the joints, promoting endurance, and being suitable for all fitness levels.

Neither is objectively better; it depends on individual goals, fitness levels, and preferences. Some might find a combination of both to be most effective.

CRAFTING THE PERFECT CARDIO ROUTINE

Creating an effective cardio routine requires understanding your goals, current fitness level, and any limitations you might have. Here are steps to guide you:

1. **Define Your Goals:** Are you aiming for fat loss, endurance enhancement, or both?
2. **Choose Your Mode:** From running, cycling, swimming, to dance, pick what you enjoy.
3. **Start Slow:** If you're new to cardio, begin with steady-state exercises to build endurance.
4. **Incorporate Variety:** Mix HIIT with steady-state workouts to prevent plateaus and keep things interesting.
5. **Listen to Your Body:** Ensure you have rest days to allow recovery and reduce the risk of injuries.
6. **Stay Consistent:** Like any fitness regimen, consistency is key. Set a schedule and stick to it.

In wrapping up, cardiovascular exercises are a potent tool in the arsenal of anyone looking to achieve a leaner physique. Whether you're sprinting in short bursts or taking long, scenic runs, the key is to keep that heart pumping. By understanding the benefits, choosing the right type for you, and crafting a tailored routine, you're on the path to not just a leaner, but a healthier you.

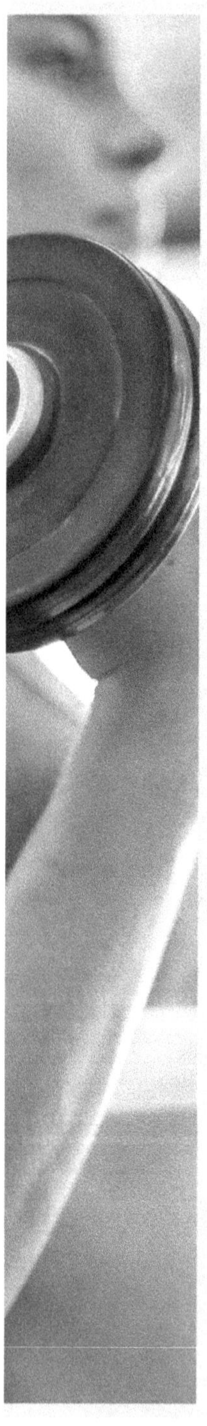

Chapter 5

STRENGTH AND RESISTANCE: SCULPTING A STRONGER CORE

MUSCLE: THE UNSUNG HERO OF METABOLISM

While cardiovascular exercises often steal the limelight in fat-loss discussions, the role of muscle in this journey is paramount. Muscles are metabolically active tissues, meaning they burn calories even when you're at rest. The more muscle mass you have, the higher your resting metabolic rate, making it easier to maintain or lose weight.

THE IMPORTANCE OF MUSCLE IN FAT METABOLISM

Muscle tissue serves as a powerhouse in our body, consuming energy even during periods of inactivity.

Here's how muscle aids in fat metabolism:

- **Increased Caloric Burn**: Muscles, when active, burn calories, and even at rest, they consume more energy than fat tissues.
- **Enhanced Insulin Sensitivity**: Muscle growth can improve insulin sensitivity, reducing the risk of type 2 diabetes and aiding in efficient nutrient absorption.
- **Support for Cardio Workouts**: Strong muscles enhance performance in cardiovascular exercises, allowing for longer and more intense workouts.

CORE-FOCUSED STRENGTH EXERCISES

A strong core goes beyond the aesthetic appeal of a toned midsection. It supports posture, reduces back pain, and aids in almost every physical activity. Here are some effective core-focused exercises:

1. **Planks**: A full-body workout that intensely targets the core. Variations include side planks, forearm planks, and plank leg lifts.
2. **Russian Twists**: Sitting on the floor, lean back slightly and twist your torso to touch the ground beside you, holding a weight or dumbbell.
3. **Leg Raises**: Lying flat on your back, raise your legs without bending the knees and then lower them without letting them touch the ground.
4. **Mountain Climbers**: Starting in a plank position, bring one knee towards the chest and then switch, mimicking a running motion.
5. **Deadlifts**: While primarily a back and leg exercise, deadlifts engage the core, especially the lower back, when performed correctly.

THE MYTH OF SPOT REDUCTION

One of the most enduring myths in fitness is the idea of spot reduction – the belief that you can target fat loss in specific areas of the body by doing exercises that target those areas. The truth is, fat loss occurs throughout the body based on genetics, hormones, and other factors. While core exercises will strengthen and tone the abdominal muscles, they won't specifically burn belly fat. For visible abs or a toned core, a combination of overall body fat reduction through diet and exercise, along with strength training, is essential.

In conclusion, while the journey to a leaner midsection often emphasizes cutting calories and cardio, strength, and resistance training, especially focused on the core, is an indispensable component. By understanding the metabolic advantages of muscle, incorporating core-strengthening exercises, and dispelling myths, you're paving the way for a stronger, leaner, and healthier you.

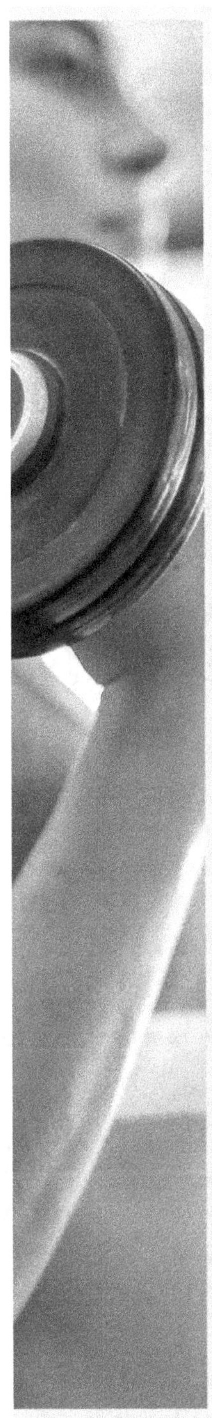

Chapter 6

FLEXIBILITY AND MINDFULNESS: THE ROLE OF YOGA AND PILATES

THE GRACE OF FLEXIBILITY

Flexibility is often the unsung component of fitness, overshadowed by strength and endurance. Yet, it plays a pivotal role in overall health, ensuring joint health, reducing injury risk, and enhancing functional movement in daily life.

THE IMPORTANCE OF MUSCLE IN FAT METABOLISM

1. **Injury Prevention**: Flexible muscles and tendons are less prone to injuries, especially during dynamic movements or strength training exercises.
2. **Improved Posture**: Flexibility in the spine and core muscles can correct postural imbalances, reducing strain on the lower back.
3. **Enhanced Range of Motion**: Flexible joints move more efficiently, aiding in strength training and aerobic exercises.
4. **Reduced Muscle Soreness**: Improved flexibility can lead to less muscle tightness and reduced post-workout soreness.

YOGA AND PILATES FOR CORE STRENGTH AND MENTAL WELL-BEING

While both yoga and Pilates emphasize flexibility, core strength, and mindfulness, they approach these goals differently:

- **Yoga**: Originating in ancient India, yoga combines physical postures, breathing techniques, and meditation. It not only enhances flexibility but also builds muscle strength, especially in the core. The meditative aspects of yoga promote mental well-being, reducing stress and enhancing focus.
- **Key Poses for Core**: Boat Pose, Plank, Crow Pose, and Warrior III.
- **Pilates**: Developed in the early 20th century by Joseph Pilates, this method focuses on core strength, flexibility, and overall body balance. Pilates exercises often use specific apparatus, but many movements can be done mat-based.
- *Key Exercises for Core*: The Saw, The Hundred, Scissor Kicks, and Teaser.

Both yoga and Pilates emphasize the mind-body connection, promoting not just physical strength but also mental resilience and clarity.

BREATHING EXERCISES FOR STRESS REDUCTION

Breath is the bridge between the mind and body. Both yoga and Pilates emphasize the importance of conscious breathing:

- **Pranayama (Yoga Breathing)**: Techniques like Anulom Vilom (alternate nostril breathing) and Kapalbhati (skull shining breath) not only enhance lung capacity but also promote relaxation and mental clarity.
- **Pilates Breathing**: In Pilates, the emphasis is on lateral thoracic breathing, where inhalation expands the ribcage sideways, and exhalation engages the core. This type of breathing supports the core-focused movements of Pilates.

Regular practice of these breathing exercises can reduce stress, lower blood pressure, and improve focus.

In wrapping up, the journey to a leaner midsection and overall well-being isn't just about how much you can lift or how fast you can run. It's also about how gracefully you can move and how mindfully you can breathe. Integrating flexibility and mindfulness practices like yoga and Pilates into your routine can offer a holistic approach to fitness, ensuring a balanced, strong, and serene you.

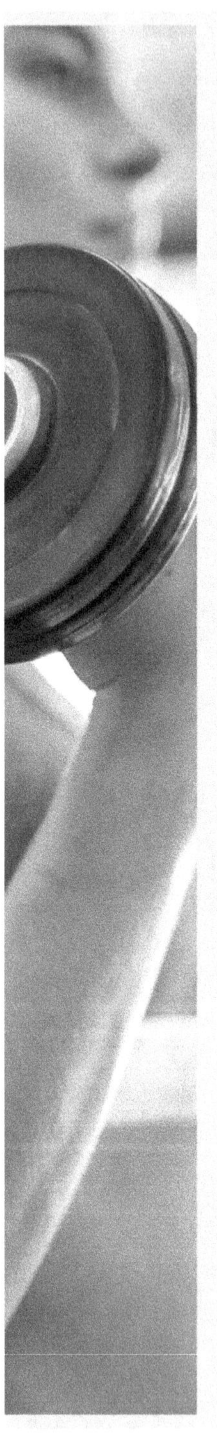

Chapter 7

SLEEP AND RECOVERY: THE UNSUNG HEROES OF FAT LOSS

THE SILENT REGENERATORS

In the cacophony of workout routines, diet plans, and fitness hacks, the quiet, restorative powers of sleep and recovery often go unnoticed. Yet, they are the unsung heroes, the backstage workers, ensuring that the body not only adapts but thrives.

THE SCIENCE OF SLEEP AND WEIGHT MANAGEMENT

Sleep isn't just a passive state of rest; it's when the body gets industrious, repairing, rejuvenating, and rebalancing. Here's how sleep influences weight:

1. **Hormonal Balance**: Lack of sleep can disrupt the balance of hunger-regulating hormones - ghrelin (which signals hunger) and leptin (which signals fullness). Sleep deprivation can increase ghrelin and decrease leptin levels, leading to increased appetite and calorie consumption.
2. **Insulin Sensitivity**: Chronic sleep deprivation can lead to reduced insulin sensitivity, increasing the risk of type 2 diabetes and making weight management challenging.
3. **Metabolism and Resting Metabolic Rate**: Prolonged sleep deprivation can slow down metabolism, reducing the number of calories burned at rest.

4. **Decision Making:** A well-rested brain is better equipped to make healthier food choices, resist temptations, and stick to workout routines.

IMPORTANCE OF RECOVERY IN MUSCLE DEVELOPMENT

Muscles aren't built in the gym; they're built during the recovery phase. When we exercise, especially strength training, tiny tears form in our muscles. Recovery allows these tears to heal and the muscles to grow stronger. Key points include:

1. **Protein Synthesis**: Recovery periods, especially sleep, are when the body synthesizes proteins to repair and build muscle tissue.
2. **Reduced Risk of Injuries**: Without adequate recovery, muscles and tendons can become chronically fatigued, increasing the risk of injuries.
3. **Mental Recovery**: Just as the body needs rest, the mind does too. Recovery periods prevent burnout and keep motivation levels high.

TIPS FOR A REJUVENATING SLEEP ROUTINE

Achieving quality sleep is both an art and a science. Here are some tips to cultivate a sleep-conducive environment:

1. **Consistency is Key:** Try to go to bed and wake up at the same time every day, even on weekends.
2. **Create a Sleep Sanctuary**: Ensure your bedroom is dark, quiet, and cool. Consider using blackout curtains, earplugs, or a white noise machine if needed.
3. **Limit Screen Time**: The blue light from phones, tablets, and computers can interfere with the production of melatonin, a sleep-inducing hormone. Aim to disconnect at least an hour before bed.
4. **Mind Your Diet:** Avoid large meals, caffeine, and alcohol before bedtime. These can disrupt sleep or reduce its quality.

5. **Establish a Pre-sleep Ritual**: Activities like reading, taking a warm bath, or practicing gentle stretches can signal the body that it's time to wind down.

In conclusion, while the world celebrates the hustle, it's the quiet hours of rest and recovery that truly shape our fitness journey. Recognizing the profound impact of sleep and recovery on weight management and overall well-being is the first step. Prioritizing them is the game-changer. As you journey towards a leaner you, remember to rest, recover, and rejuvenate.

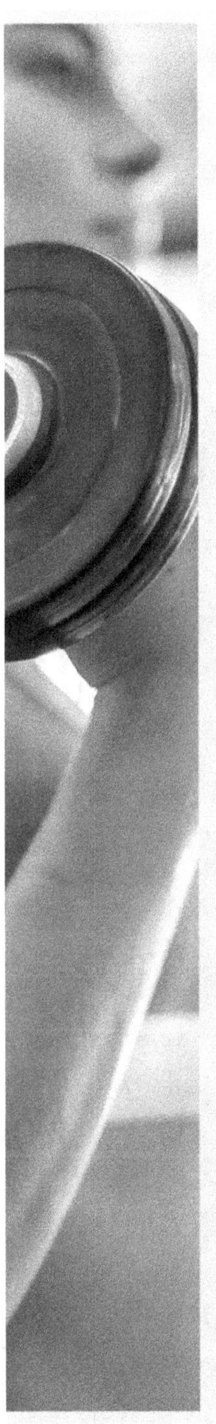

Chapter 8

HYDRATION HABITS: DRINKING YOUR WAY TO A LEANER MIDSECTION

THE LIQUID LIFELINE

Water, the essence of life, plays a pivotal role in our health and well-being. Beyond quenching thirst, it's a vital component in the intricate machinery of our body, influencing everything from cellular function to weight management.

THE SCIENCE BEHIND HYDRATION AND WEIGHT LOSS

Water isn't just a passive bystander in our weight loss journey; it's an active participant. Here's how hydration aids in shedding those pounds:

1. **Boosting Metabolism**: Drinking water can temporarily boost metabolic rate. Studies have shown that drinking about 500ml of water can increase metabolism by 10-30% for an hour.
2. **Appetite Suppression**: Often, our bodies confuse thirst with hunger. Drinking water before meals can create a sense of fullness, leading to reduced calorie intake.
3. **Enhanced Physical Performance**: Proper hydration ensures optimal muscle function and reduces the risk of cramps, allowing for more effective workouts.
4. **Detoxification**: Water aids in flushing out toxins and waste products, ensuring smooth kidney function and reducing water retention.

BEST PRACTICES FOR DAILY HYDRATION

To harness the benefits of hydration, it's essential to incorporate healthy water-drinking habits:

1. **Start Your Day Right**: Begin your morning with a glass of water to kickstart your metabolism and replenish any overnight losses.
2. **Infuse Your Water**: If plain water doesn't appeal to you, add slices of fruits, cucumbers, or herbs like mint for a refreshing twist.
3. **Mind Your Workouts**: Ensure you're well-hydrated before, during, and after exercise. Intense workouts, especially in hot climates, can lead to significant fluid loss.
4. **Use Technology**: There are numerous apps available that remind you to drink water and track your daily intake.
5. **Listen to Your Body**: While aiming for 8 glasses a day is a general guideline, individual needs vary. Pay attention to your body's signals and adjust accordingly.

In wrapping up, water, in its simplicity, holds the power to transform our health and weight loss journey. By understanding its multifaceted role, debunking myths, and adopting healthy hydration habits, you're not just paving the way to a leaner midsection but also ensuring optimal health and vitality. Drink up and thrive!

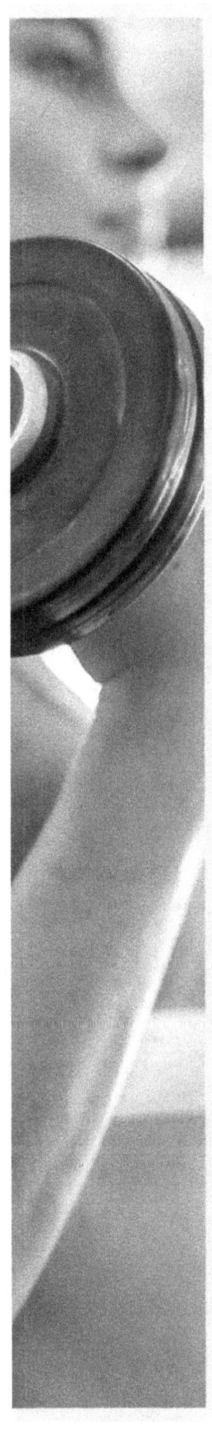

Chapter 9

STRESS AND THE BELLY FAT CONNECTION

THE SILENT SABOTEUR

In the modern world, stress has become an almost constant companion for many. While occasional stress can be a motivator, chronic stress, especially when not managed, can have profound implications on our health, particularly in weight management and fat accumulation around the midsection.

HOW CORTISOL AFFECTS WEIGHT

Cortisol, often dubbed the "stress hormone," is released by the adrenal glands in response to stressors. While it serves essential functions, chronic elevated levels can wreak havoc on our bodies:

1. **Appetite Regulation**: Cortisol can stimulate appetite and increase cravings for sugary, fatty foods, leading to overconsumption.
2. **Fat Storage**: Elevated cortisol levels can promote fat storage, especially in the abdominal area. This visceral fat, as discussed earlier, is metabolically active and poses significant health risks.
3. **Muscle Breakdown**: Chronic high cortisol can lead to muscle protein breakdown, reducing lean muscle mass and subsequently slowing down metabolism.
4. **Insulin Resistance**: Prolonged stress can lead to imbalances in blood sugar levels, promoting insulin resistance and increasing the risk of type 2 diabetes.

MINDFULNESS AND MEDITATION
TECHNIQUES FOR STRESS REDUCTION

Recognizing the detrimental effects of chronic stress, it's crucial to find effective ways to manage and mitigate it. Mindfulness and meditation have emerged as powerful tools:

1. **Basic Mindfulness Meditation**: Sit in a comfortable position, focus on your breath, and bring your attention to the present moment. When your mind wanders, gently bring it back to your breath.
2. **Guided Imagery**: Listen to guided recordings that lead you through a series of calming visuals, helping you relax and center.
3. **Progressive Muscle Relaxation**: Tense and then relax each muscle group in your body, starting from your toes and working your way up.
4. **Body Scan Meditation**: Mentally scan your body from head to toe, noting sensations and releasing tension.
5. **Loving-kindness Meditation**: Send out feelings of love and well-being, first to yourself and then to others, fostering positive emotions.

THE LINK BETWEEN MENTAL WELL-BEING
AND PHYSICAL HEALTH

The mind-body connection is profound. Mental well-being doesn't just influence our thoughts and emotions but has tangible effects on physical health:

1. **Immune Function**: Chronic stress and poor mental health can suppress the immune system, making the body more susceptible to infections.
2. **Heart Health**: Stress and anxiety can increase blood pressure and the risk of heart diseases.
3. **Digestive Health**: Mental well-being affects gut health, leading to issues like indigestion, bloating, and even irritable bowel syndrome.
4. **Longevity**: Positive mental well-being has been linked to longer, healthier lives.

In conclusion, while the journey to a leaner midsection often focuses on diet and exercise, the role of mental well-being is paramount. Recognizing the profound impact of stress, especially its influence on belly fat, and adopting practices like mindfulness and meditation, can pave the way for holistic health. As the saying goes, "It's not the load that breaks you, it's the way you carry it." Equip yourself with the tools to manage stress, and watch your path to a leaner, healthier you become clearer and more achievable.

Chapter 10

STAYING THE COURSE: MOTIVATION, TRACKING, AND CELEBRATING WINS

THE MARATHON, NOT THE SPRINT

The journey to a leaner midsection and holistic well-being is akin to running a marathon, not a sprint. It's a long-term commitment, punctuated with highs and lows, successes and setbacks. The key to reaching the finish line? Staying motivated, tracking progress, and celebrating every win, no matter how small.

SETTING AND MAINTAINING REALISTIC GOALS

1. **SMART Goals**: Ensure your goals are Specific, Measurable, Achievable, Relevant, and Time-bound. Instead of "I want to lose weight," aim for "I want to lose 10 pounds in the next three months."
2. **Break It Down**: Large goals can be daunting. Break them into smaller, more manageable milestones. This makes the journey less overwhelming and provides frequent moments of achievement.
3. **Stay Flexible**: Life is unpredictable. There might be times when you're unable to stick to your plan. Instead of getting disheartened, adjust your goals and move forward.

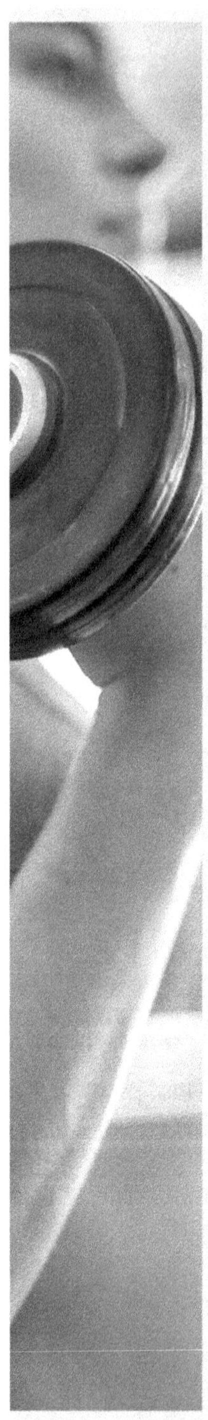

TOOLS FOR TRACKING PROGRESS

In the age of technology, numerous tools can help you stay on track:

1. **Fitness Apps**: Apps like MyFitnessPal, Fitbit, and Lose It! allow you to log your meals, workouts, and track weight loss.
2. **Wearable Tech**: Fitness trackers and smartwatches can monitor steps, heart rate, sleep patterns, and more, giving you insights into your health.
3. **Journaling**: The traditional pen and paper approach can be therapeutic. Documenting your journey, feelings, and achievements can provide motivation and clarity.
4. **Photos**: Taking regular progress photos can be a visual testament to your journey, showcasing changes that might not always reflect on the scale.

THE IMPORTANCE OF CELEBRATING SMALL VICTORIES

1. **Boosts Motivation**: Every time you acknowledge and celebrate a win, you reinforce the positive behavior that led to that success, making it more likely you'll repeat it.
2. **Builds Confidence**: Recognizing your achievements, however small, can boost self-esteem and confidence, essential components for long-term success.
3. **Provides Perspective**: Celebrating small wins helps you focus on the journey rather than just the end goal. It's a reminder that every step, no matter how tiny, is a move in the right direction.
4. **Creates Momentum**: Each small victory can act as a stepping stone, propelling you forward with renewed vigor.

In wrapping up, remember that the journey to a leaner you is unique. It's a tapestry woven with individual challenges, strengths, setbacks, and successes. While the destination—a healthier, leaner midsection—is undoubtedly important, so is the journey. By setting realistic goals, tracking your progress, and celebrating every victory, you're not just working towards a physical transformation but also cultivating resilience, determination, and self-love. Stay the course, embrace the journey, and watch yourself evolve, both inside and out.

Conclusion

THE HOLISTIC APPROACH TO A LEANER, HEALTHIER YOU

THE SYMPHONY OF WELLNESS

As we reflect upon the journey traversed through these ten chapters, it becomes evident that the path to a leaner midsection and holistic well-being is not a solitary endeavor. It's a symphony, where each component—nutrition, exercise, sleep, hydration, mental well-being—plays its unique note, contributing to the harmonious melody of health.

INTEGRATING KNOWLEDGE INTO ACTION

1. **Understanding the Anatomy**: Recognizing the difference between visceral and subcutaneous fat sets the foundation, allowing us to approach weight loss with clarity and purpose.
2. **Nutrition's Nuances**: It's not just about eating less but eating right. Balancing macronutrients and choosing nutrient-dense foods fuels our body optimally.
3. **Energy Dynamics**: Grasping the concept of caloric balance—energy in vs. energy out—empowers us to make informed decisions about our diet and activity levels.
4. **The Power of Movement**: Cardiovascular exercises and strength training, each with its unique benefits, work in tandem to sculpt our physique and boost metabolism.

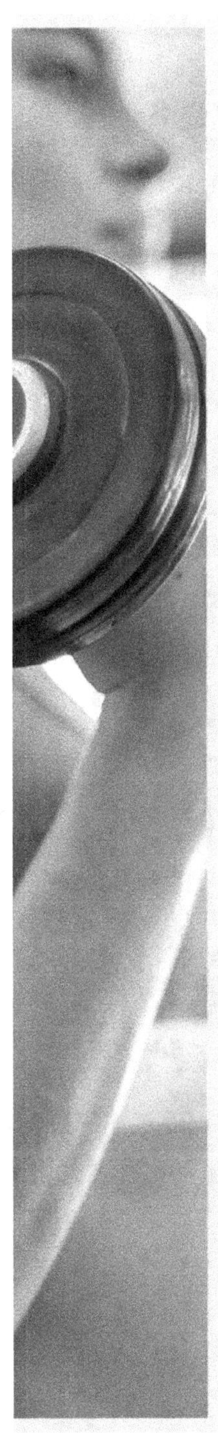

5. **Flexibility and Mindfulness**: Beyond physical strength, the grace of movement and the serenity of the mind play pivotal roles in our overall well-being.

6. **Rest and Recovery**: In the hustle to achieve, we learned the importance of pause—how sleep and recovery are integral to muscle development and overall health.

7. **Hydration's Role**: Water, the essence of life, emerged not just as a thirst quencher but as a vital player in weight management.

8. **Mental Well-being's Influence**: Stress, and its physiological manifestations, highlighted the profound mind-body connection, emphasizing the need for mental balance in a physical journey.

9. **Staying Motivated**: Setting goals, tracking progress, and celebrating victories, both big and small, ensure we stay the course, even when the going gets tough.

THE JOURNEY AHEAD

As we close this book, it's essential to remember that knowledge, while powerful, is only the beginning. The real magic happens when we integrate this knowledge into our daily lives, making consistent, informed choices that align with our goals.

The journey to a leaner, healthier you is not linear. There will be peaks and valleys, moments of triumph, and days of struggle. But with every step, every choice, you're not just moving closer to your physical goals but also cultivating resilience, self-awareness, and a deeper connection with yourself.

Embrace this journey with an open heart, a curious mind, and the unwavering belief that you are capable of incredible transformations. Here's to a leaner, healthier, more vibrant you. The journey has only just begun.